C000051499

Belinda Thompson

About the Book:

Children's Book
Written by: Belinda Thompson
Illustrated by: HH-PAX
Title: Embracing Our Differences

"Embracing Our Differences" is a story about a Hispanic three-year-old boy who goes to school for the very first time and is suffering from a rare medical condition called Dravet Syndrome. Although the syndrome can affect every aspect of a child's life, Matias is fighting every day to live a fun, energetic, and meaningful life with a condition that his tomorrow is not promised. Even at the tender age of three, Matias is a trooper with the will to fight every day. His adoring soul touches everyone around him, and his heart became a magnet to his nurse Belinda Thompson, who developed a special bond with a child who she believes is God's most precious gift. This book was inspired by the lack of awareness and education about the Dravet Syndrome in our community and Public School System and written to spread attention to epilepsy and its numerous forms. The title was inspired due to us all being born different. Every individual has a special gift and/or talent regardless of their medical condition. When we as a whole can appreciate the reality of our differences, we can then learn to embrace them.

FOREWORD

As a registered nurse for 35 years, I have worked in many diverse clinical settings. During the past 10 years, I have worked in the Pediatric Primary Care and Pediatric Specialty Ambulatory Care Clinics. During a casual conversation with my friend Belinda Thompson, who is a new Registered Nurse, she spoke of one of her young patients. She is so excited about her position as a Professional Registered Nurse caring for a three-year old patient with Dravet Syndrome. Our discussion proceeded and Belinda asked "Gwen, do you know what Dravet Syndrome is"? I was so embarrassed, particularly since I work in the Pediatric Neurology Clinic; I delayed for a couple of moments and gradually answered, "NO".

I would like to thank Belinda Thompson for not only bringing awareness and educating me about Dravet Syndrome; but also, for sharing her personal experiences pertaining to the care of patients with this disorder. Her book, "Embracing Our Differences" will bring awareness and education to the Public Health, Medical, and Nursing Community about Dravet Syndrome. In the wake of my discovery, this is an exceptionally unprecedented and uncommon issue that causes uncontrollable seizures. I now understand the physical, emotional, and financial impact on caregivers and families.

Belinda Thompson has brought great insight of what it's like living with Dravet Syndrome and the fundamental resiliency in providing care to her patient who she describes to be "God's most precious gift". I am excited for the journey she is about to embark upon and wish her much success in her future endeavors.

Nurses not only care for their patients but also show them they deserve care and that they truly want to help improve their quality of life. It has always been a desire to be a part of that process—to care for others and hopefully help improve their quality of life, both physically and mentally. I am grateful for the knowledge I have given Belinda thus far, both in nursing and in her personal life. My hope is that the integration of the two will allow her to evolve into the healthcare professional that she ultimately wants to become. I am elated to have been a part of her process in writing "Embracing Our Differences".

Gwendolyn Mike, MPH, BSN, RN
Nurse Manager
Jackson Memorial Hospital

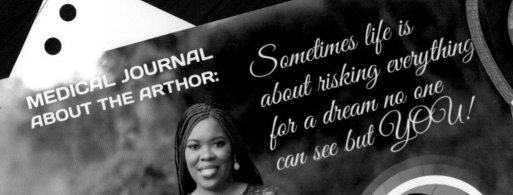

MEDICAL JOURNAL
ABOUT THE ARTHOR:

Sometimes life is about risking everything for a dream no one can see but YOU!

Belinda Thompson, on the surface, is a focused–driven individual who inspires to be an elite Healthcare Professional with a multifaceted scope of learning and instruction in the domain of business administration, nursing, human services, health information technologist, and now AUTHOR. She resides in the Sunshine State of Florida and views herself as a "pioneer" who takes pride in knowing that some of the best leaders are great followers. As such, she has engaged in many healthy and professional mentorships with individuals who she considered to be much wiser and who could push her to the next level both personally and professionally. But more than an attentive individual, Ms. Thompson is a person who is sincere and earnestly tries to influence and empower others to higher levels in their life; whose opinion is highly sought after, and whose judgement is respected and trusted. Ms. Thompson, developed a passion for writing her very first children's book when she accepted a nursing assignment of a child with a debilitating medical condition called Dravet Syndrome. Although, in the profession of nursing, she never heard of this condition in her studies, which propelled her to do research and study the condition. Frightened at first, Belinda was on for the challenge. The bond that she shares with the child is remarkable and she will always cherish the moments they share.

Embracing Our Differences

NOTES

DEDICATION:

This book is in memory of my angel:
"Daddy" (Lee Chester Peterson aka LC)

I dedicate this book to the parents of Matias Jimenez:
Michelle & Jorge Jimenez

To all the children with Dravet Syndrome and to the many caregivers who provide care for a child that suffers from any type of epilepsy/ or any other medical condition; "Always remember that you are beautiful and special to the world".

ACKNOWLEDGEMENTS

A special thanks to Integrity Health Services, Broward-County School Board and the staff of Silver Shores Elementary for providing medical and academic services to Matias Jimenez and his caregivers. Your tireless work and efforts for Matias empowered me to be inspired and create the very First Children's Book Edition of Dravet Syndrome. It is my hope that other parental figures of any type of epilepsy and/or medical condition be inspired and uplifted by the contents of "Embracing Our Differences".

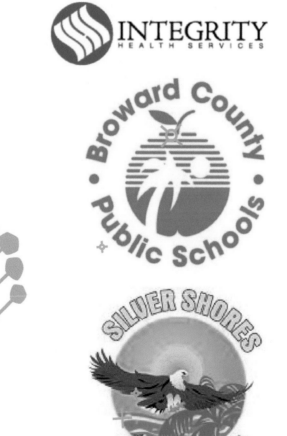

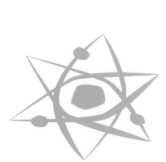

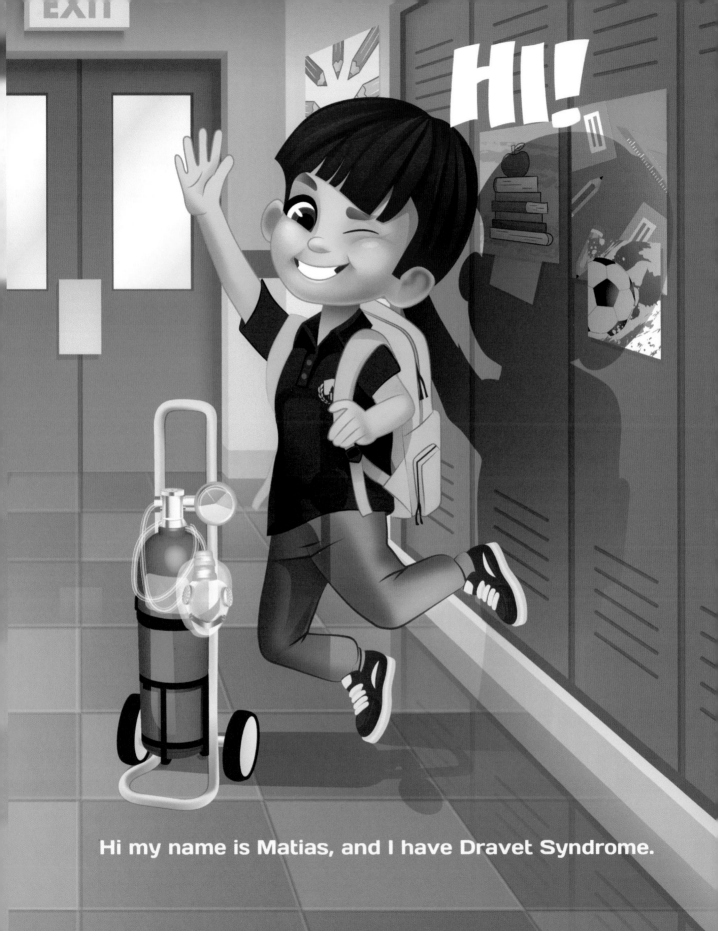

Hi my name is Matias, and I have Dravet Syndrome.

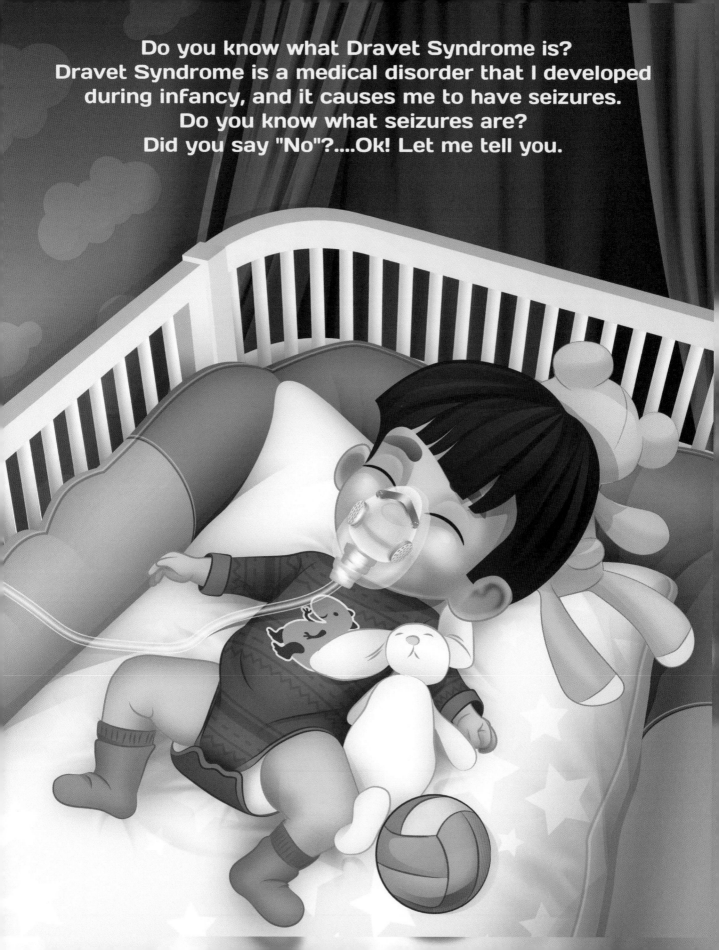

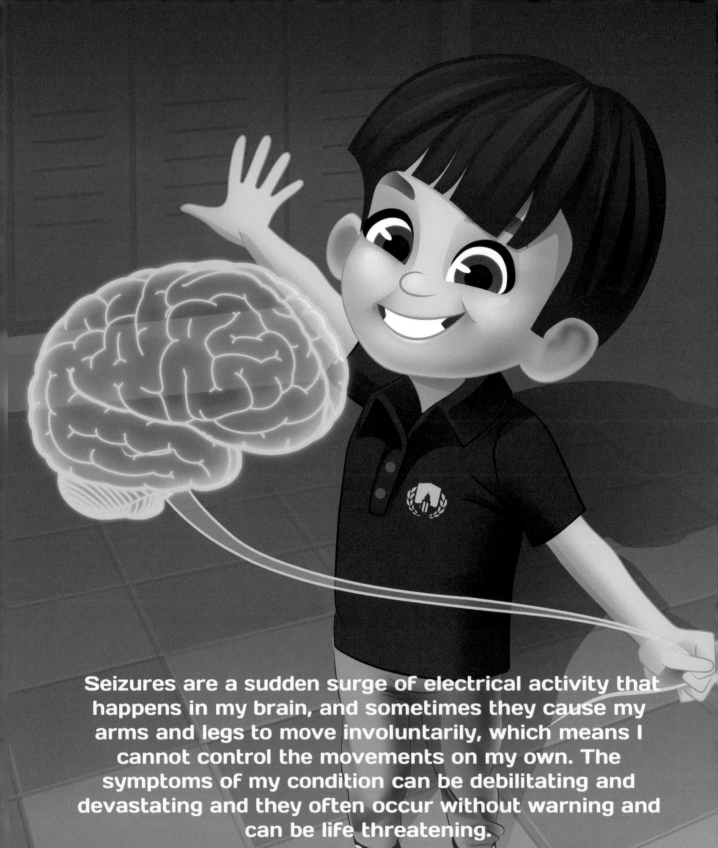

Seizures are a sudden surge of electrical activity that happens in my brain, and sometimes they cause my arms and legs to move involuntarily, which means I cannot control the movements on my own. The symptoms of my condition can be debilitating and devastating and they often occur without warning and can be life threatening.

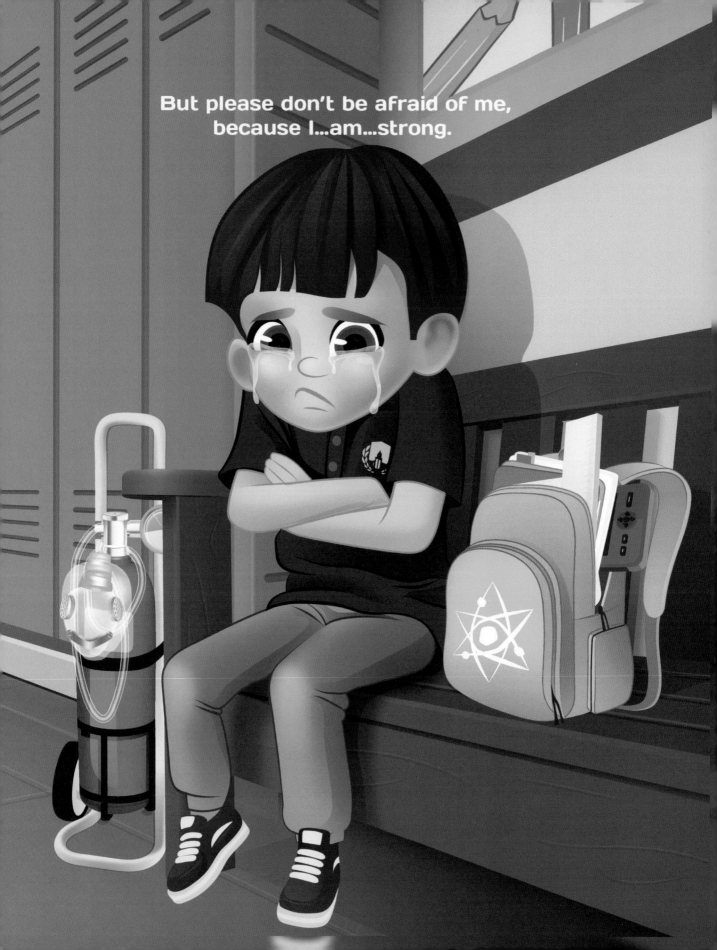

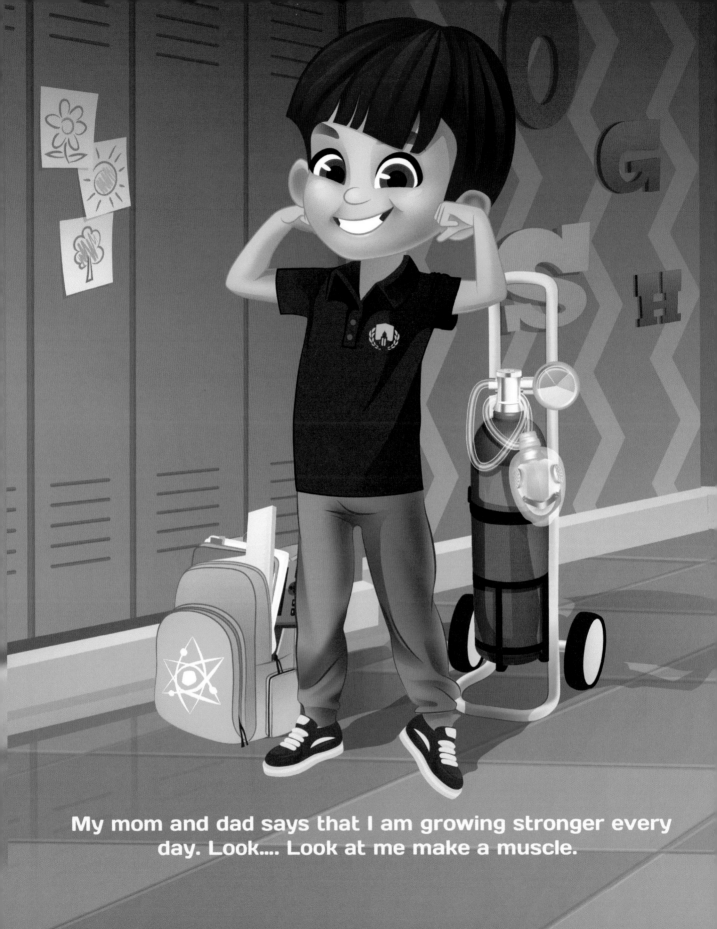

My mom and dad says that I am growing stronger every day. Look.... Look at me make a muscle.

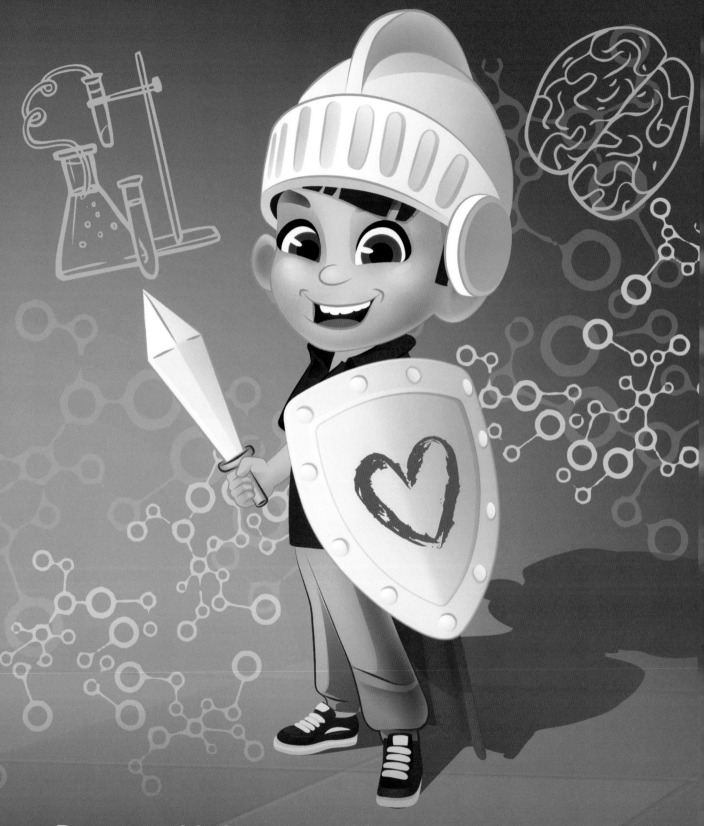

Do you want to know something cool? I am a warrior
and I will fight every day to keep a smile on your face.

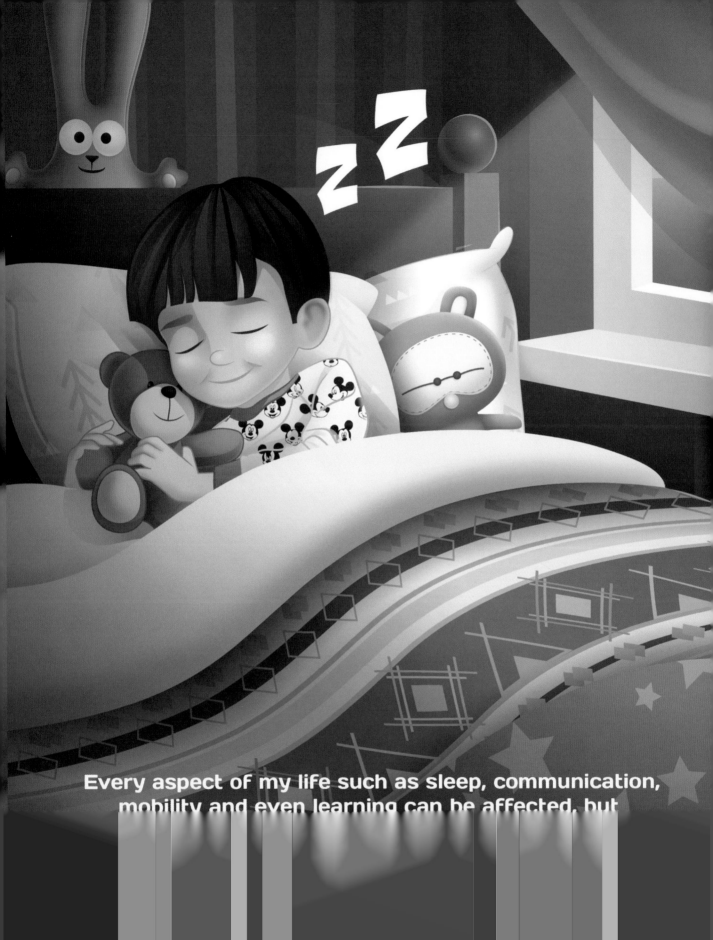

Every aspect of my life such as sleep, communication, mobility and even learning can be affected, but

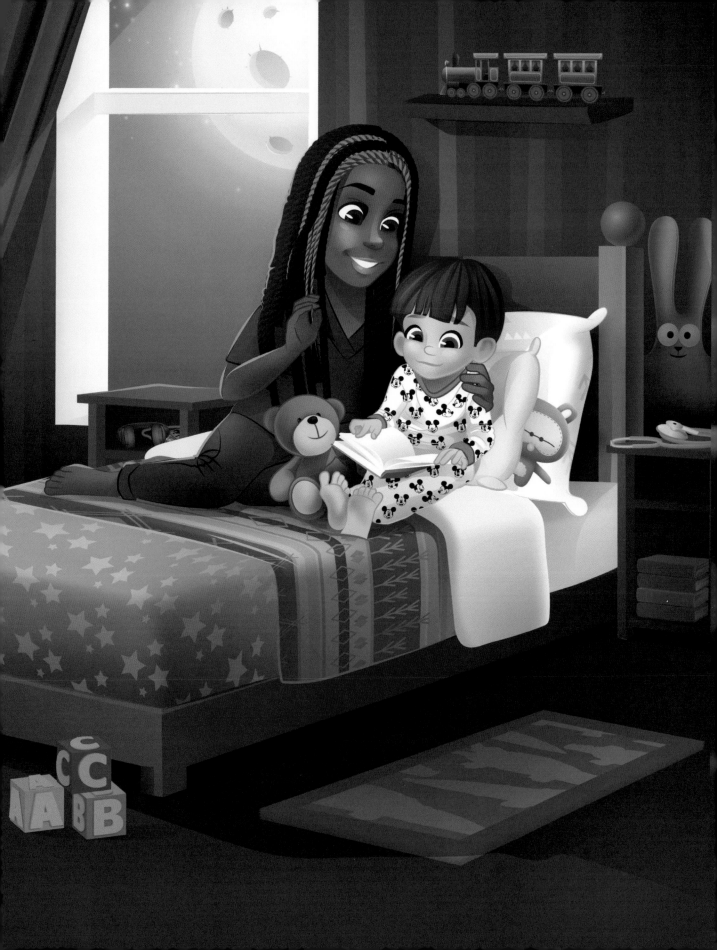

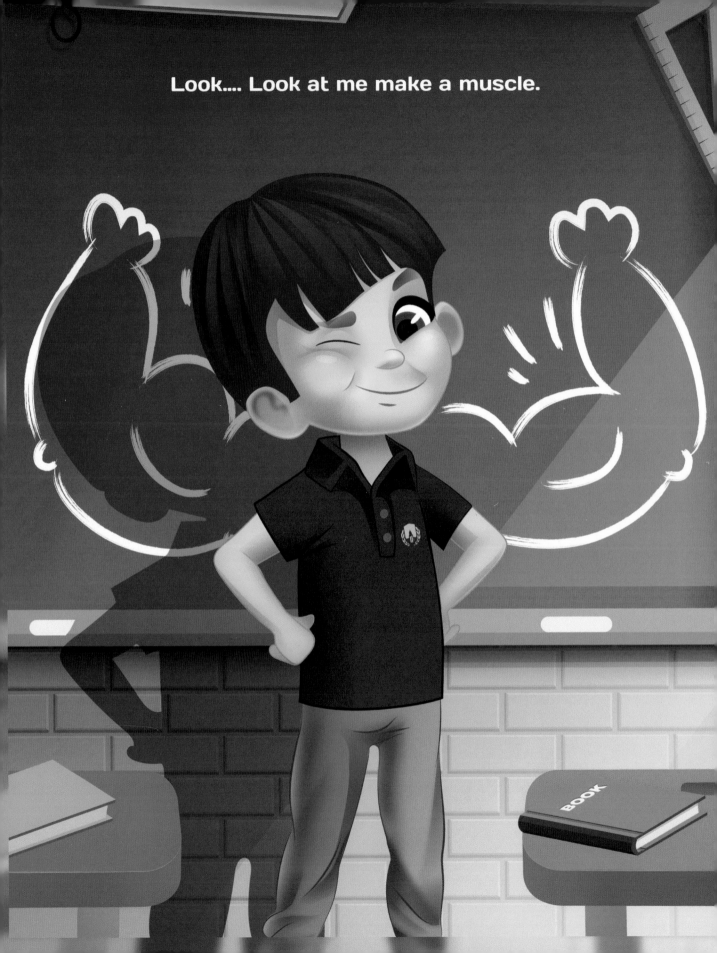

I love to play with puzzles.

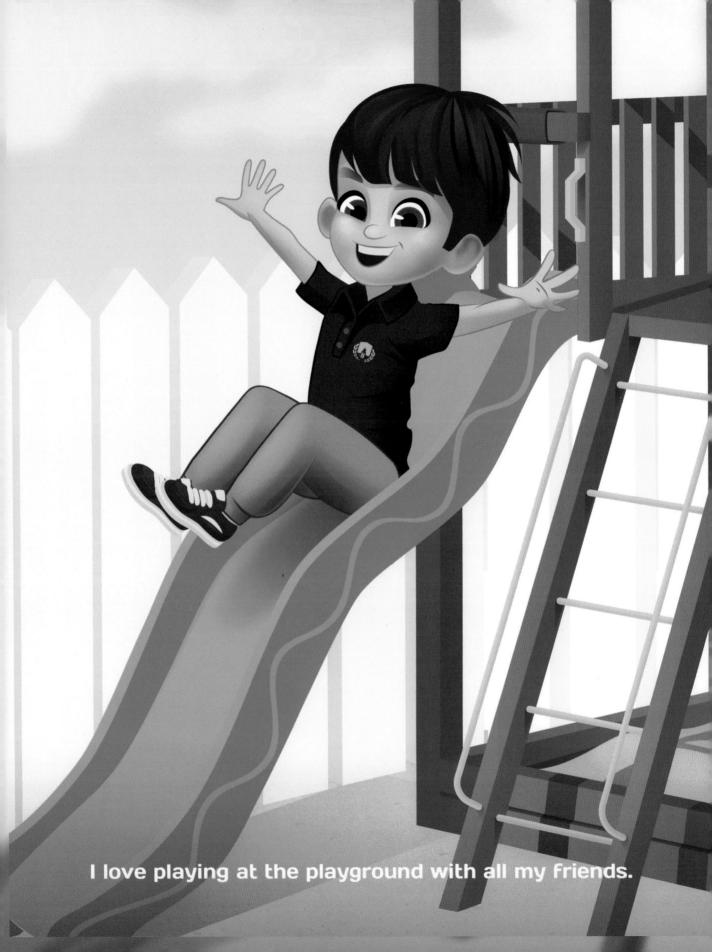

I love playing at the playground with all my friends.

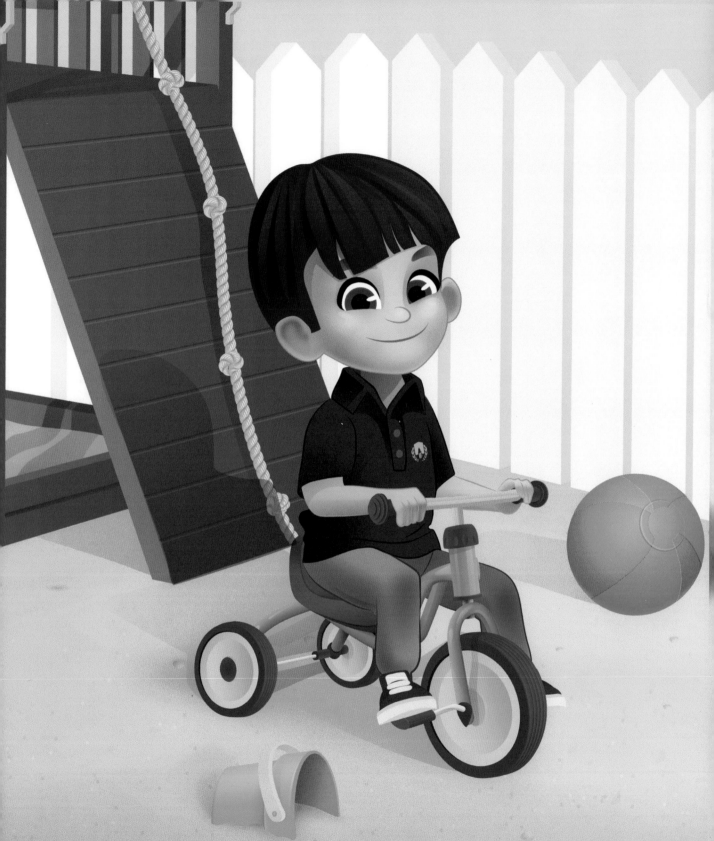

Oh, and singing with all my friends is my most favorite part of the day.

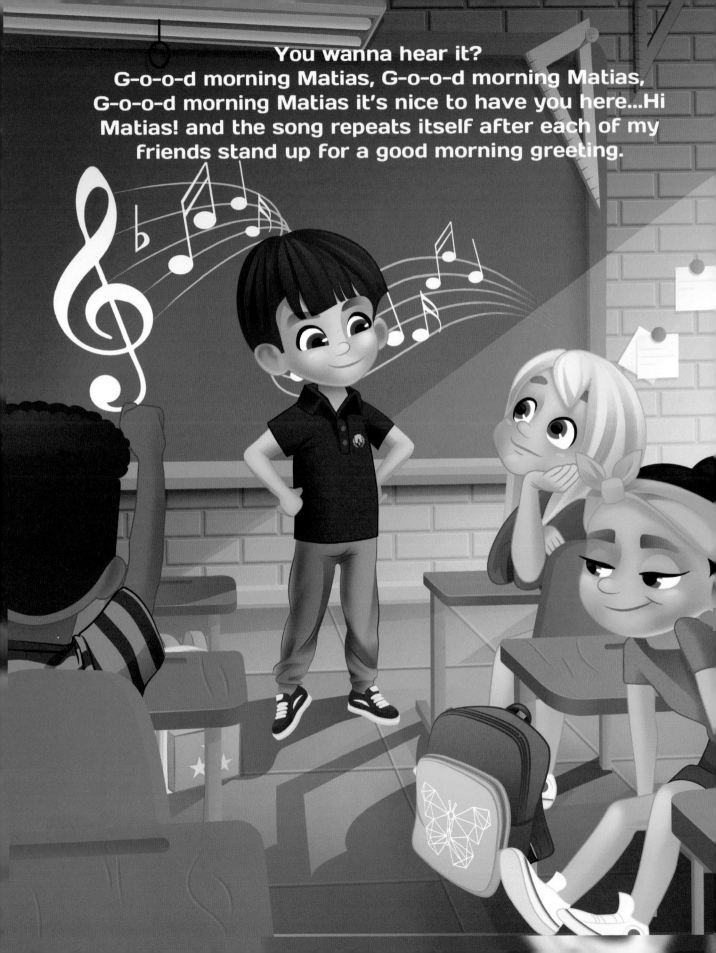

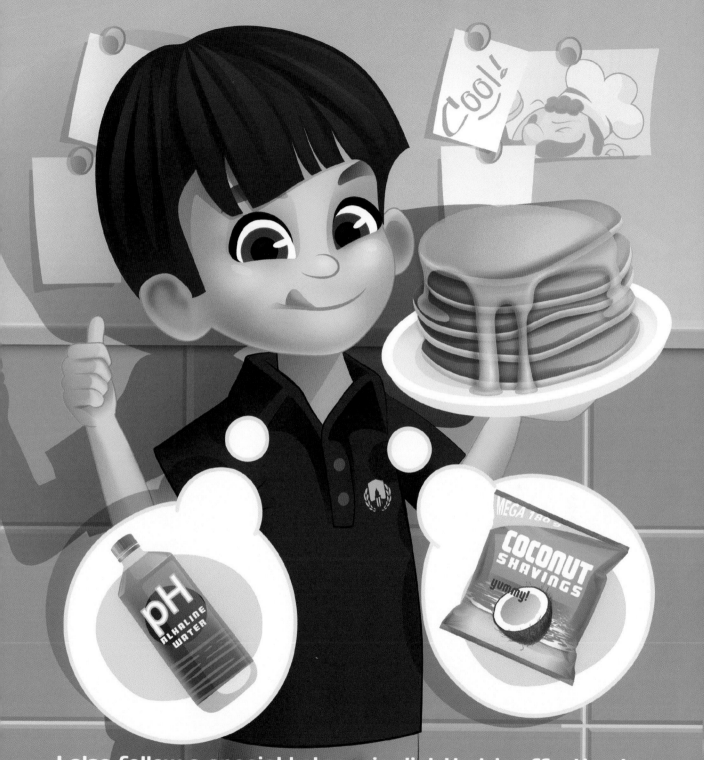

I also follow a special ketogenic diet that is effective in managing my symptoms. This diet also helps me have less seizures.

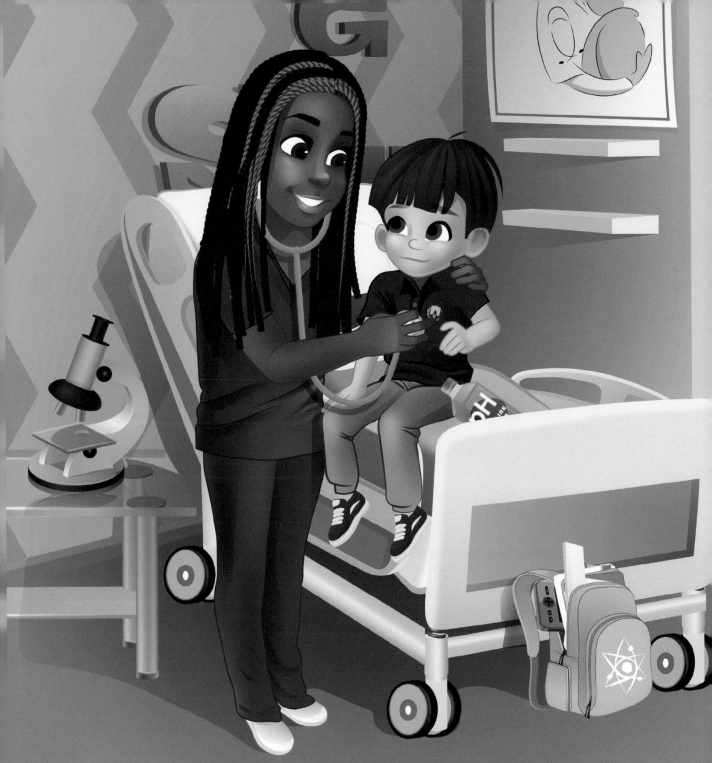

When I am at school, I have a special nurse all for me. She takes really good care of me. She monitors me every day and she even has a stethoscope to listen to my heart and lungs.

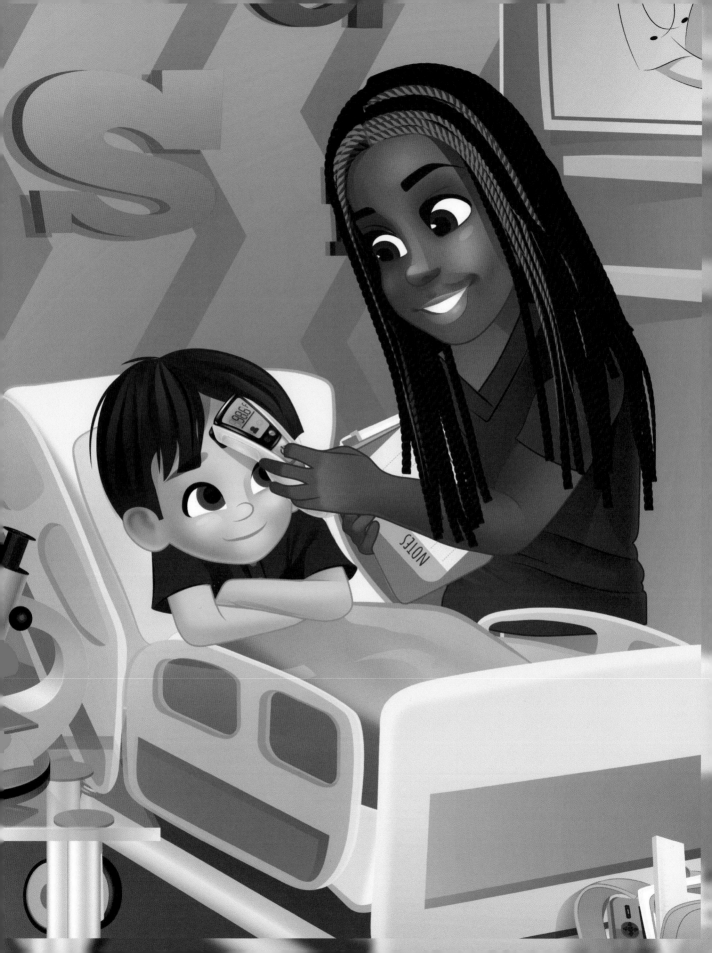

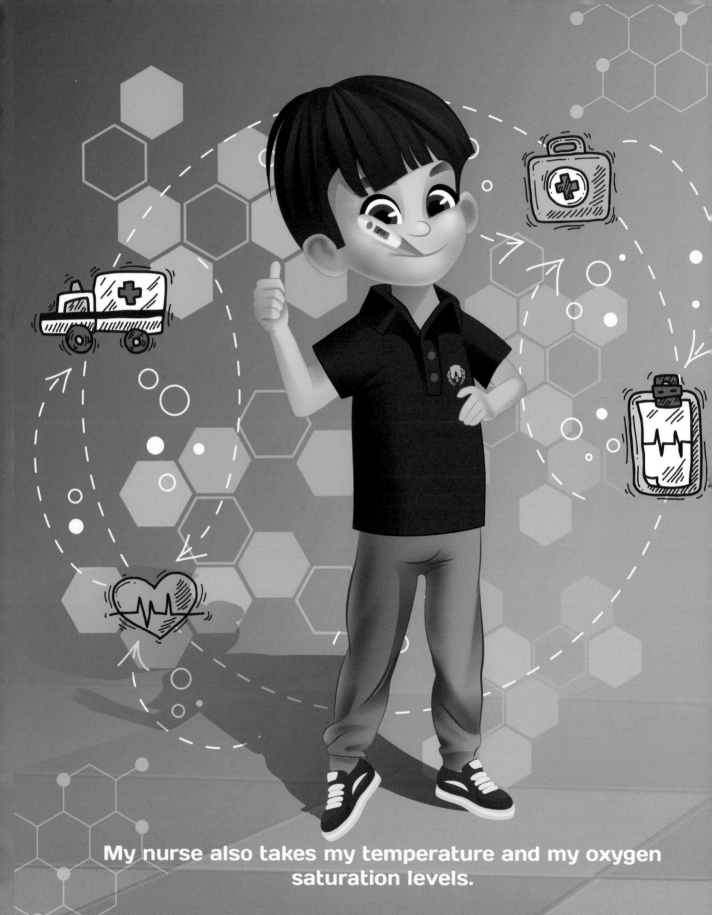

My nurse also takes my temperature and my oxygen saturation levels.

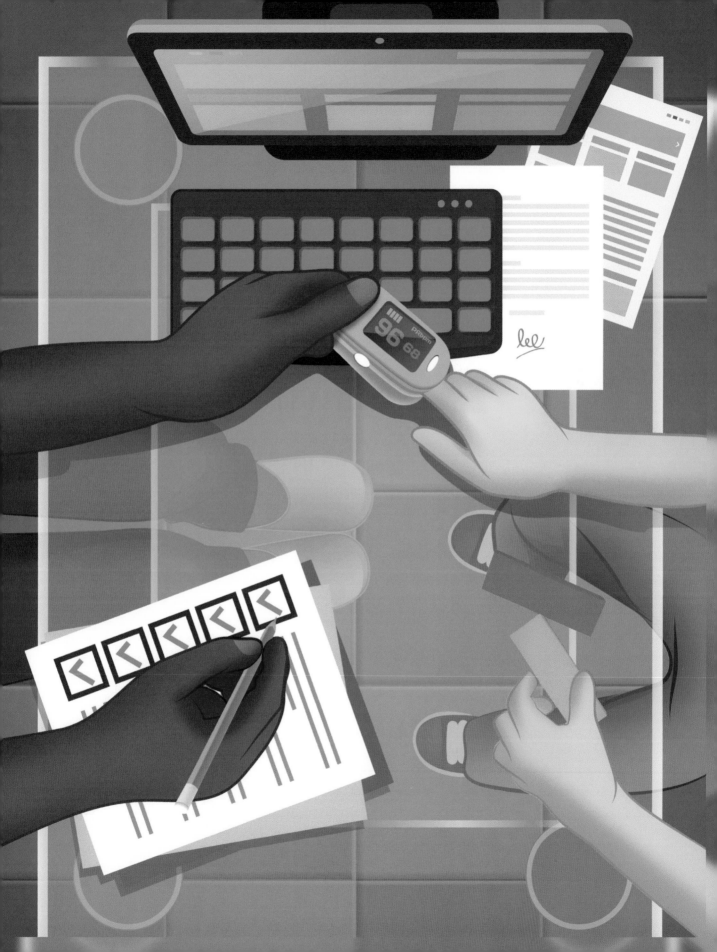

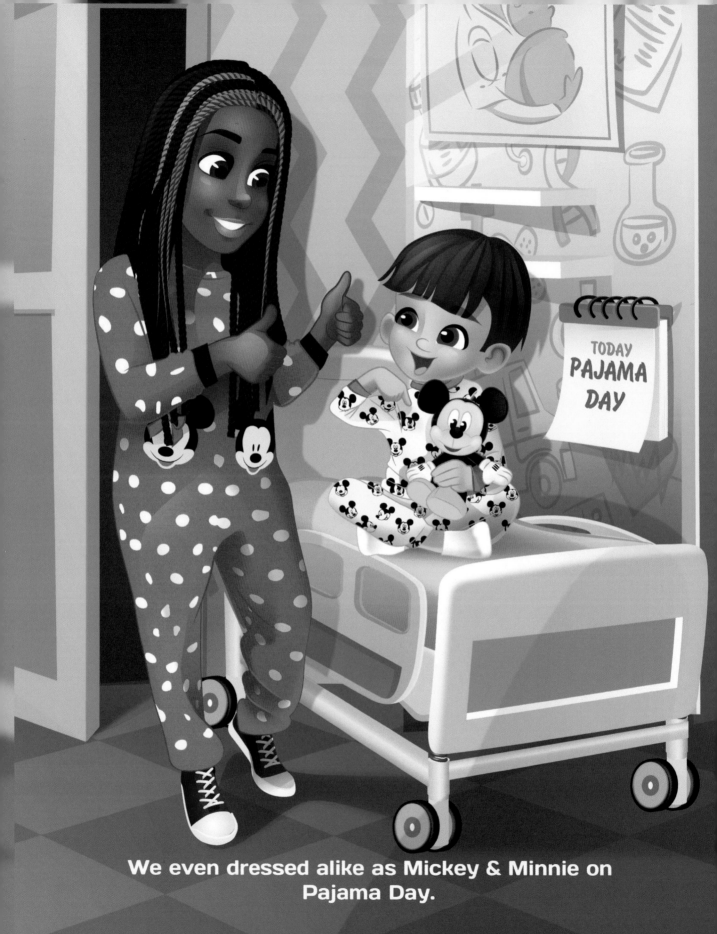

We even dressed alike as Mickey & Minnie on
Pajama Day.

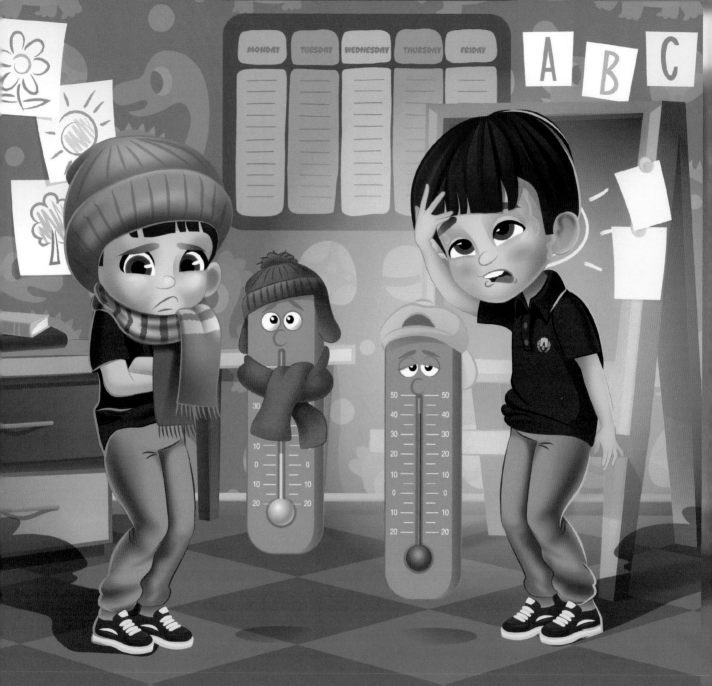

My nurse also makes sure that I avoid any triggers that may cause a seizure. She makes sure that I don't experience any sudden or quick changes to my environment. This could be a quick change in temperature (hot to cold), overexertion, overexcitement, overheating, stress, bright flashing lights and loud noises.

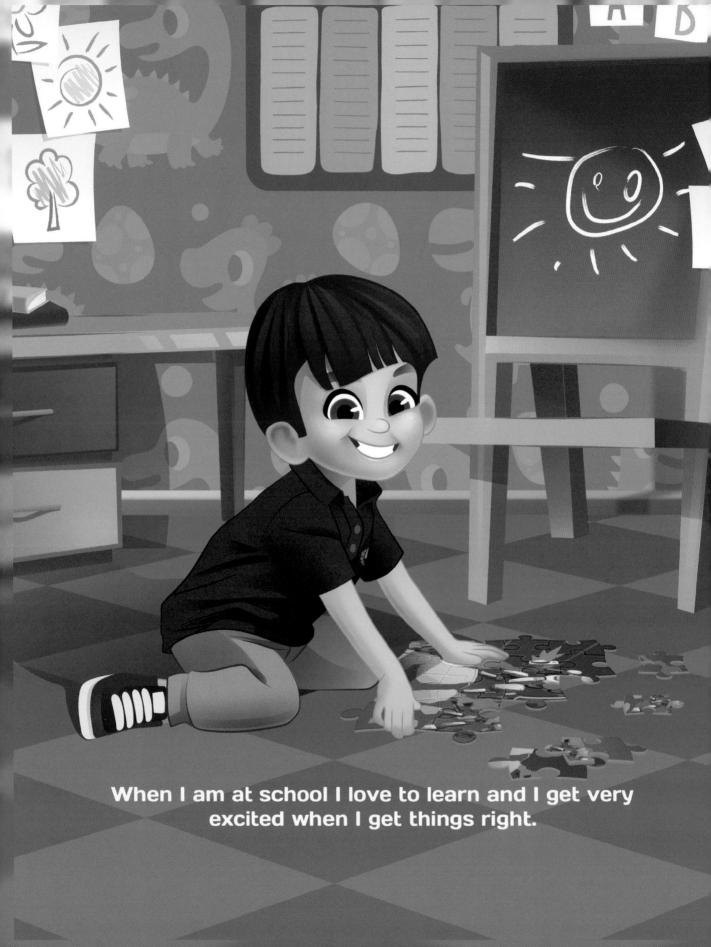

When I am at school I love to learn and I get very
excited when I get things right.

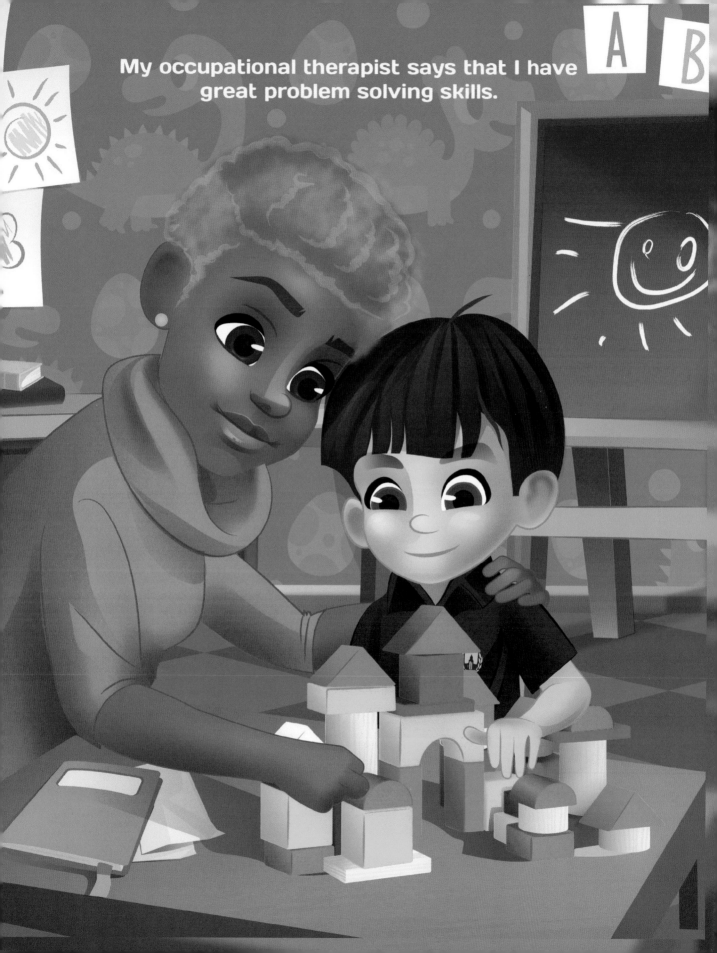

My occupational therapist says that I have great problem solving skills.

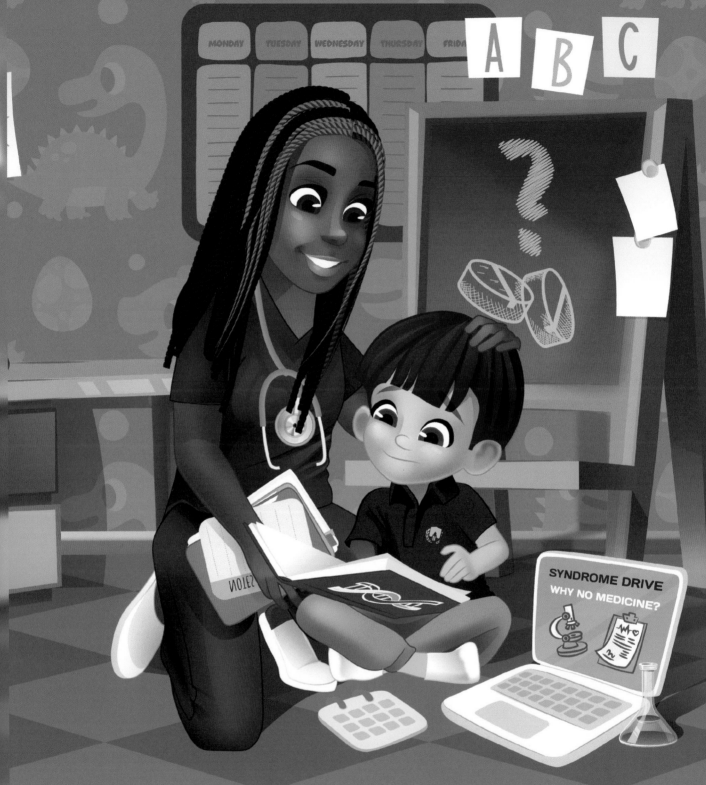

There is no cure for my disorder, but my nurse says that one day there will be!

Due to the unpredictable nature of my condition, a special medical protocol with emergency school staff was developed just for me. This team makes sure to keep me safe. I also have a really good neurologist too!

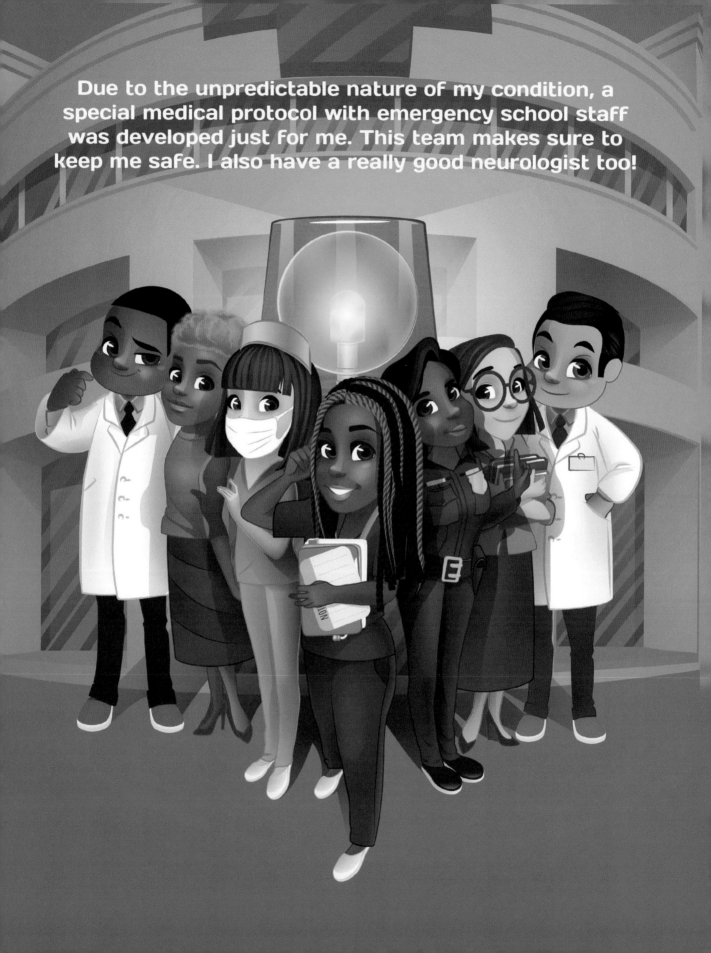

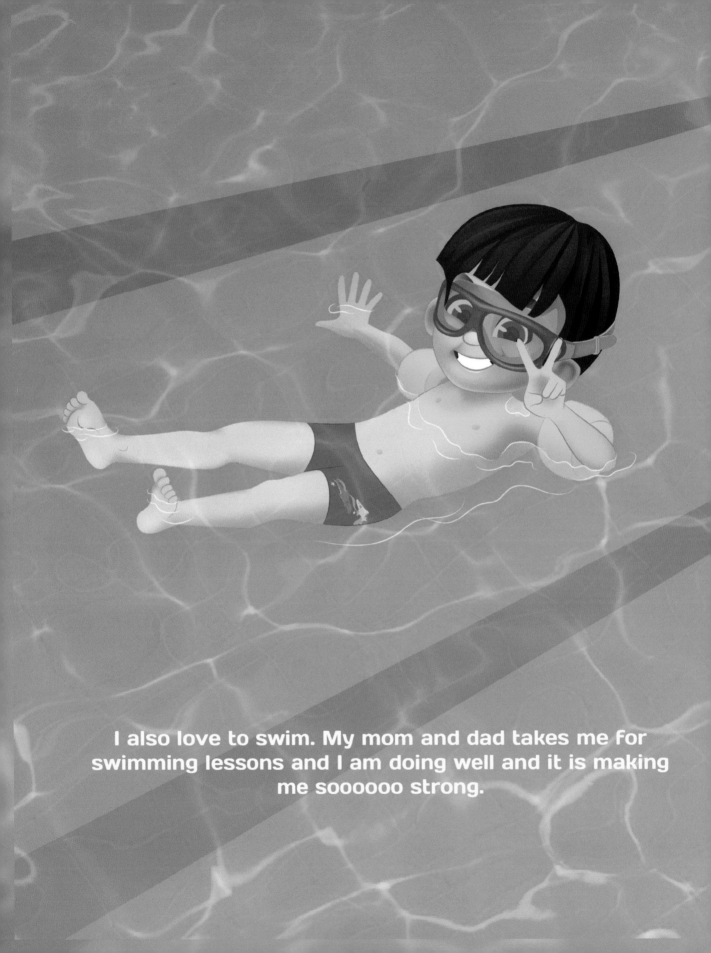

I also love to swim. My mom and dad takes me for swimming lessons and I am doing well and it is making me soooooo strong.

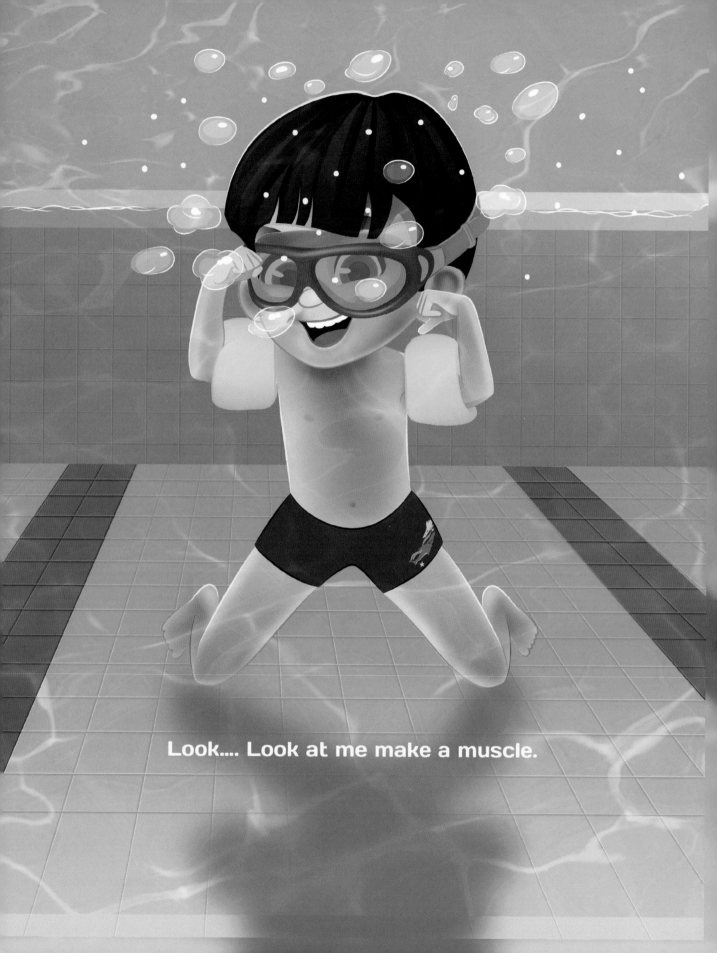

Look.... Look at me make a muscle.

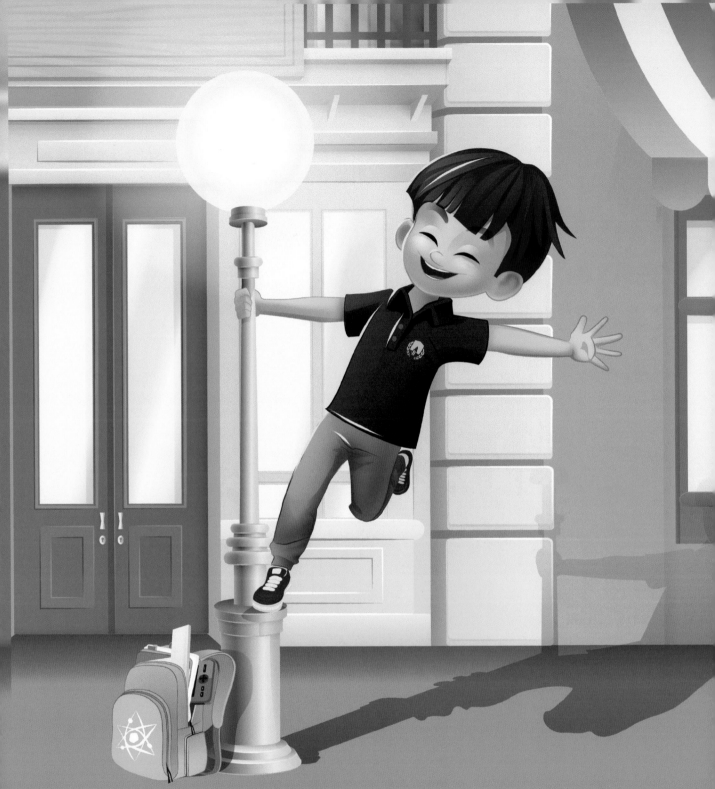

Dravet Syndrome is a medical condition that will affect me for the rest of my life, but it doesn't slow me down one bit.

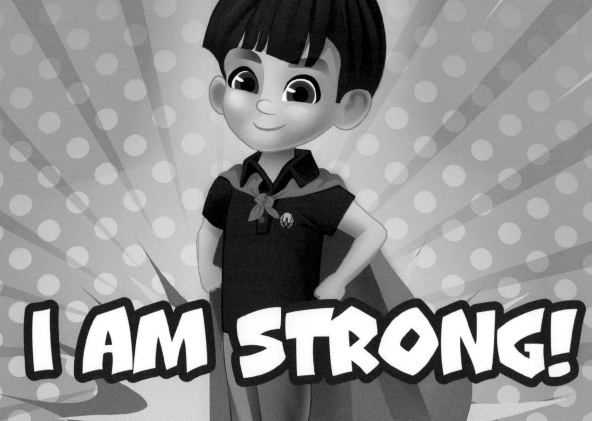

I AM STRONG!

I may have dravet syndrome but I...am...strong!
Can you make a muscle?

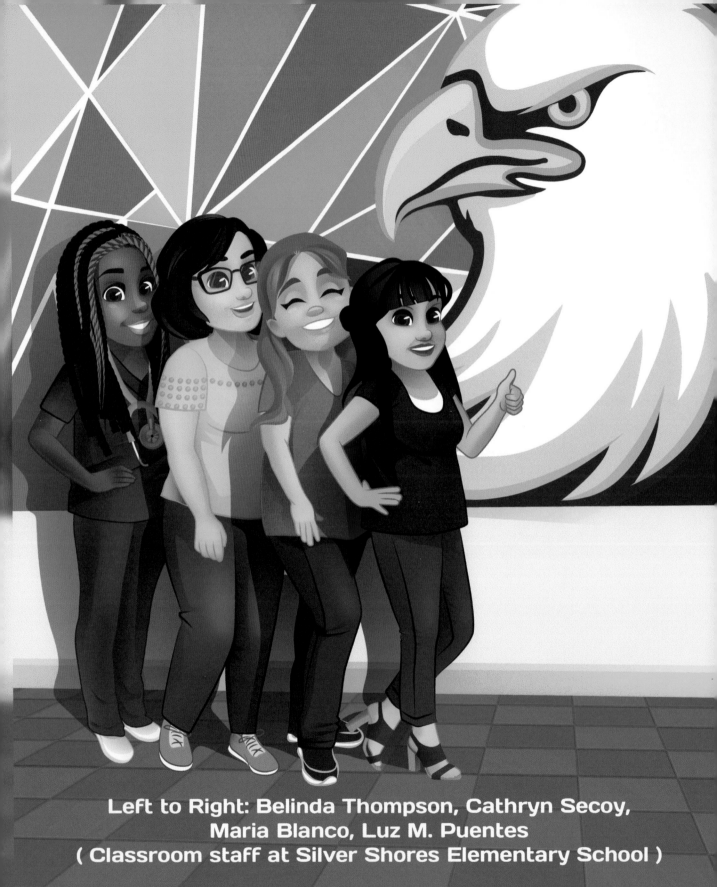

Left to Right: Belinda Thompson, Cathryn Secoy,
Maria Blanco, Luz M. Puentes
(Classroom staff at Silver Shores Elementary School)

WORD BANK

1. **Dravet Syndrome**- a rare, catastrophic, lifelong form of epilepsy that begins in the first year of life with frequent and/or prolonged seizures.

2. **Epilepsy (also called Seizure Disorder)**- a neurological disorder marked by sudden recurrent episodes of sensory disturbances, loss of consciousness, or convulsions, associated with abnormal electrical activity in the brain.

3. **Debilitating**- (of a disease or condition) making someone very weak.

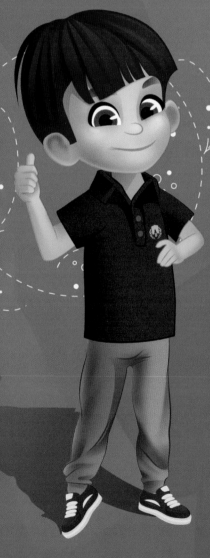

4. **Strong**- having the power to move heavy weights or perform other physically demanding task. Just like Matias ability to fight Dravet Syndrome!

5. **Warrior**- a brave or experienced soldier or fighter.

6. **Embrace**-accept or support (a belief, theory, or change) willingly and enthusiastically.

7. **Different**- not the same as another or each other; unlike in nature, form, or quality.

8. **Afraid**- feeling fear or anxiety; frightened. Worried that something undesirable will occur or be done.

9. **Neurologist**- a specialist in the anatomy, functions, and organic disorders of nerves and the nervous system.

10. **Ketogenic diet**- a high-fat, adequate-protein, low-carbohydrate diet that in medicine is used primarily to treat difficult-to-control epilepsy in children.

11. **Research**- the systematic investigation into and study of materials and sources in order to establish facts and reach new conclusions.

EMBRACING
OUR DIFFERENCES

About the Book:

"Embracing Our Differences" is a story about a Hispanic three-year-old boy who goes to school for the very first time and is suffering from a rare medical condition called Dravet Syndrome. Although the syndrome can affect every aspect of a child's life, Matias is fighting every day to live a fun, energetic, and meaningful life with a condition that his tomorrow is not promised. Even at the tender age of three, Matias is a trooper with the will to fight every day. His adoring soul touches everyone around him, and his heart became a magnet to his nurse Belinda Thompson, who developed a special bond with a child who she believes is God's most precious gift. This book was inspired by the lack of awareness and education about the Dravet Syndrome in our community and Public School System and written to spread attention to epilepsy and its numerous forms. The title was inspired due to us all being born different. Every individual has a special gift and/or talent regardless of their medical condition. When we as a whole can appreciate the reality of our differences, we can then learn to embrace them.

AUTHOR: BELINDA THOMPSON
ILLUSTRATOR: HH-PAX

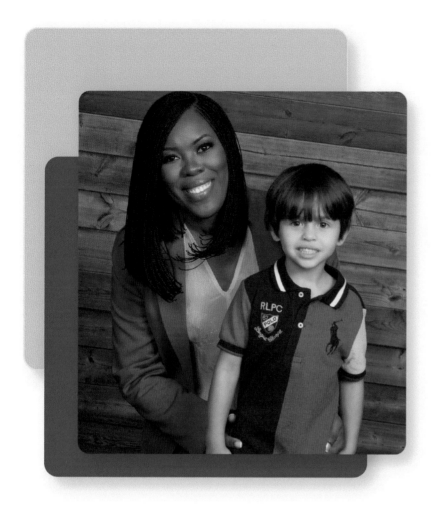

Thank you for sharing the experience of
Embracing Our Differences: Living with Dravet Syndrome.

We hope you enjoyed reading, as much as we enjoyed creating it.
Thank you for your support.

With Sincere Thanks,
Belinda & Matías

Thank You

Printed in Great Britain
by Amazon

59569788R20022